I0104002

EYES WIDE OPEN

Parenting (and Life) Manifestos for the21st Century

By John Breeding, PhD

All rights reserved, no part of this publication may be reproduced by any means, electronic, mechanical, or photocopying, documentary, film, or otherwise without prior permission of the publisher.

Published by:
Chipmukapublishing
PO Box 6872
Brentwood
Essex
CM13 1ZT
United Kingdom
http://www.chipmunkapublishing.com
Proof-read by Lucy Abbott
Copyright © 2007 John Breeding

We see the world not as it is, but as we are.
--An ancient Talmudic adage, also attributed to Anais Nin

In a dark time, the eye begins to see.
--Theodore Roethke, 1963

PREFACE

Eyes Wide Open is an effort to shed some light on the amazing and seemingly unlimited capacity of our species to live and act from a place of denial and unreality. It seems we humans are intensely vulnerable to conditioning, and that large numbers of us misperceive reality and act in destructive ways as a result. I attempt to explain how this happens and offers a few thoughts on a way out. The book consists of two parts. Book 1, *A 21st Century Manifesto for Parenting*, is a practical confrontation of some things parents must face about our highly distressed society in order to protect their children. Book 2, *Eyes Wide Open*, is a sequel, confronting the fact that protecting our own individual children is not enough, that without significant change in the way humans govern the world, our children will not have a future. This little book tries to crack a chink in the colossus of denial and ignorance, the notion being, to paraphrase the great songwriter, Leonard Cohen, that the crack is where the light gets in.

Table of Contents

BOOK 1

Scott Nearing and the Need for a Manifesto 9

Bo Lozoff and Not Doing 13

A 21st Century Manifesto for Parents 15

The Protections 16

The Commitment 29

BOOK 2

A Second 21st Century Manifesto for Parents 31

On Seeing 34

A Primer on Conditioning 42

From Eyes Wide Open to A Culture of Denial: An Awful Transmutation 45

Denial, Oppression, and Claims to Virtue 54

The New Intrusion Initiative 59

Psychiatry and Militarism: A World in Peril 62

Seeing (or Not) the Truth 67

Conclusion 71

References 77

About the Author 79

BOOK 1

Scott Nearing and the Need for a Manifesto

Sin City No More? Why Las Vegas is the face of America's future.
-Cover, US News & World Report, June 11, 2001

> We were reasonably successful in freeing ourselves from the four besetting evils of a competitive, industrialized social pattern: from greed for things (including money and gadgets) and from power to push around our fellow human beings; from the hurry and noise connected with the drive to get ahead of other people; from the anxiety and fear which are inevitable accompaniments of the struggle for wealth and power; from the multiplicity, complexity, and frustrating confusion which result from the crowding of multitudes of people into small areas.
> -Scott Nearing, 1972. *The Making of a Radical,* p. 214.

Born in 1883, Scott Nearing devoted his life to challenging the destruction caused by Western Civilization and its attendant primary value on profit for a few, via systematic conditioning of competitive, acquisitive and consumptive attitudes. Scott and his wife, Helen, also observed in their lifetime that the American urban and suburban family had virtually disappeared as a

social unit and as a social force. With everybody busily working in the system, and children turned over
to the forces of compulsory education, the rhythms, routines and regularities of home living have become much less significant in children's lives.

I agree with the Nearings that Western Civilization, with its clear and consistent emphasis on militarism, competition, industrialism, materialism, and profit for the few at the expense of the many is costing us all. Clearly it is hurting our children. If health is an indicator of the quality of an individual's relationship with his or her environment, then increases in chronic illnesses and obesity in children clearly reflect our society's failure. If literacy and psychological well-being are indicators of the quality of children's development, then growing numbers of illiterate, "learning disabled" and otherwise "psychiatrically afflicted" children clearly show the failure of our civilization. If relaxed confidence, trust and safety are indicators of the quality of a child's development, then we are failing many. If fraud and deceit, drugs, violence and imprisonment of adults are indicators of failed character development, then the way we raise young people in Western Civilization is a disaster.

A definitive indicator of the quality of a civilization is in the care of its young. Since mothers are the primary caretakers of children, a rational civilization must, by any measure, value mothers over militarism. In the same vein, the care of children depends on available caring fathers; therefore, a rational civilization must value the health and well-being of its men over militarist expansion and corporate profit. These priorities are not and never have been true of Western Civilization.

Since the care of children depends on adequate availability of basic needs, the financial wellbeing of working families must always be a priority over the excess wealth of a minority and excess military might. This too is not and never has been true of Western Civilization. What is true is the reality of what I call parental oppression-a state of hardship due to the systematic neglect and mistreatment of families, parents and children alike, for the sake of the power and greed inherent in an exploitative approach to people and the world.

Parenting has always been a difficult challenge, but it is especially hard today because of the lack of real support in our society, and because of the deleterious effects on community, in the form of alienation and separation, which were wrought by the priorities of militarist, industrialist and capitalist civilization. Parenting is hard not because parents are doing a bad job; in fact, parents are doing heroically well under the circumstances. As an example of this, we may for the first time have a small, but significant cohort of young people who are being raised with an attitude of complete respect from their parents. This in itself is a wonderful and remarkable thing. Nevertheless, the decline of Western Civilization as we know it may be seen in the tremendous stress and neglect from which so many of our children are suffering. Denying this only supports its perpetuation. Facing it, however, allows for the possibility of real help for our children in the form of everyday heroic action by parents.

Bo Lozoff and Not Doing

In his latest book, *It's A Meaningful Life*, Bo Lozoff, director of the Human Kindness Foundation, puts into perspective the apparent negative orientation of so many religious precepts with the following statement:

> In fact, most of the great spiritual commandments, precepts, and teachings throughout history have been merely guidelines for what we should stop. Most of the Ten Commandments start with "Thou shalt not"; the Buddhist precepts and Hindu Yamas and Niyamas start with "non"-as in non-killing, non-stealing, non-lying. Contemporary people
> have often complained that the ancient teachings are too negative, but the reason they are phrased negatively is that there really isn't anything to do in order to realize the Divine Presence, the natural Holiness life offers. We merely have to stop thinking and acting in ways that are harmful or selfish or off the mark.
>
> The great teachings unanimously emphasize that all the peace, wisdom, and joy in the universe are already within us; we don't have to gain, develop, or attain them. Like a child standing in a beautiful park with his eyes shut tight, there's no need to imagine trees, flowers, deer, birds, and sky;

we merely need to open our eyes and realize what is already here, who we already are---as soon as we stop pretending we're small or unholy.

I could characterize nearly any spiritual practice as simply being: identify and stop, identify and stop, identify and stop. Identify the myriad forms of limitation and delusion we place on ourselves, and muster the courage to stop each one. Little by little deep inside us, the diamond shines, the eyes open, the dawn rises; we become what we already are. *Tat Twam Asi* (Thou Art That). (Pp. 173-4)

The following manifesto is strong. Remember that its intention is merely to protect and uncover the truth that it is good to be alive and to be with children. It may be seen as a spiritual practice, supporting us to identify and stop the obscurities of the glory of our children's, and our own, true nature.

A 21st Century Manifesto for Parents

I recognize that our society is seriously disturbed and dangerous to the well-being of my family and my children in many ways. I recognize that our society has institutionalised many obviously harmful practices as acceptable tradeoffs for the perpetuation of the dominant values of Western Civilization. This is not acceptable to me. Therefore, I vow to keep my eyes open, to educate myself, and to provide protection for my children to the best of my ability against the most grievous harms, some of which include the following.

The Protections

I will provide protection against…

… *unnecessary prenatal trauma.* We have now verified scientifically what aware mothers have always known—that babies are enormously affected by their prenatal experience. It is the responsibility of parents to see that mothers are well-nourished and protected from all forms of stress overload. It would be well to remember that some cultures actually use the prenatal time to contact the soul that is incarnating in the baby to find out their purpose for this life. Taken literally or metaphorically, this is a wonderful reminder of the perennial spiritual wisdom, reflected in the immortal words of Kahlil Gibran, "your children are not your children." We parents are the protectors and guardians of an awesome being during its years of physical and psychological development. What a glorious task!

…*unnecessary birth trauma.* We also know that the birth experience is a most powerful determinant of well-being. While some progress has been made in reclaiming this natural process from the mid-20th century extremes of medical technological control, it remains true that unnecessary drugs, use of force, and other harmful birthing practices unduly harm many mothers and babies. It is the responsibility of parents to ensure as natural and benign a birthing experience as possible. This includes protecting against separation, which can disrupt the bonding of mother and infant.

…the trauma of circumcision. This harmful, cruel and unnecessary relic, justified by cultural, religious and pseudo-scientific superstition, should be avoided.

…the trauma of in-arms deprivation. In-arms deprivation is a term coined by Jean Liedloff to characterize the effects of a very specific unmet need; the need to be carried in arms, to be held virtually all the time in the first six months of life. Many older children and adults suffer anxiety and irrational dependency because of this infant deficiency. Alternatively, many are somewhat detached and shut down, and don't even think they need physical contact and affection. What a gift for parents and children to delight in close contact and affection throughout their lives!

…the trauma of unnecessary immunizations. Vaccine proponents are recommending more and more immunizations. These include vaccines for diseases not particularly dangerous to children (e.g., chicken pox) or for which children are not generally at risk (e.g., hepatitis B). Furthermore, governments are pushing for more coercion in this area. Much is known about the dangers of various vaccines. Parents should be completely educated on this subject before making decisions which may have permanently damaging effects on

their children's lives. Those who decide some immunization is good should be especially well-informed about the vaccines they choose to have administered to their children and should be able to discern reactions. The newborns should be protected from postpartum immunization, and parents should be extremely wary about immunizations later during their infancy.

...the trauma of toxic and unhealthy foods. America's food industry is a callous and mercenary exploiter of children; the horrible effects of massive intake of processed foods, sugar and toxic substances on our children are enormous. Parents must resist this damaging influence and do everything they can to see that our children are well-nourished. At the least, this means restriction of sugar (in all its disguises), chemical additives and preservatives, fast foods and processed foods. For many, perhaps most children, this also means restriction of dairy and, for some, of other common allergenic foods such as wheat and corn. This also means reliance on fresh, whole foods, preferably organic. Plenty of water is essential, as is adequate intake of the essential fatty acids. (See the work of John Robbins, author of *Diet For A New America*, and his organization, EarthSave, for more information and support for activism on school lunches and other issues.)

...the trauma of separation from nature. What a great tragedy it is to deprive a child the experience

of hours in the natural world of earth and sky, grasses, flowers, bushes, trees, water, bugs, birds and animals of all kinds. It is so much more important that children play with dirt rather than electronic games.

…the trauma of TV and video. The average American child watches hours of electronic media every day. The deleterious effects of this practice are enormous, both direct and indirect. Directly, through its impact on central nervous system function and programming of consciousness, and indirectly through the sacrifice of time spent in more wholesome, creative activities.

…the trauma of computers. Conscious professionals are now challenging the unconscious assumption that this technology is good for young children. A useful guideline is to protect children from all involvement with computers until they are fluent in reading and cursive writing, and to limit elementary age children to 30 minutes per day.

…the trauma of a sedentary lifestyle. Movement, activity, physical play and exercise—these are essential to the healthy development of a child's body and mind.

…the trauma of compulsive busyness. Fast (and furious) may be the trend of modern western civilization, but it is not healthy. Our children need lots of relaxed down time to be alone and with

friends and family—not to be constantly entertained and stimulated, but to be allowed and encouraged to discover themselves and their world by creating and producing their own activities. A related problem is the tendency to deny children necessary experience and opportunities to learn and contribute because it is easier and quicker for parents to do it themselves. It's best for parents to take the time to let children help, even if it takes two hours to do the dishes with them instead of the 10 minutes it would take to do them yourself. Finally, my own and others' informal observation is that 90% of punishment incidents take place because of time pressure. We do yourselves and our children a favor by arranging our lives as much as possible at a slower pace.

...*the trauma of sleep deprivation.* A large percentage of Americans, including our children, are sleep deprived. Parents must protect children from being forced to accommodate to adult needs and schedules. Rhythm, routine and regularity are keys for a well-ordered life, and especially for a safe, relaxed, healthy environment in which a child can fully develop themselves. The greatest result can be achieved not just through the direct interventions, but also through the indirect effects promoted by creating a safe haven, a rich relational world, and a healthy environment.

...*the trauma of "adultism".* "Adultism" refers to the systematic mistreatment of young people by adults, simply because they are young. The key indicator is disrespect. One of the best ways for adults to assess whether they are perpetrating "adultism" on a young person is to ask themselves whether they would say the same thing in the same tone of voice, with the same facial expression, and with the same gestures to another adult that they had just communicated to a young person. It is crucially important for parents to challenge "adultism" because the effects of this form of oppression (hurt, fear, shame, and the internalised pattern of disrespect) are exactly the reason why other forms of oppression (such as racism, sexism, gay oppression) are allowed to exist. Without being systematically hurt and psychologically conditioned to be mean and disrespectful, adults would not stand for mistreatment of themselves or others.

...the trauma of emotional suppression. This one is enormously important. Humans are incredibly intelligent and sociable by nature, but when physically or emotionally hurt, the resultant distress causes us to become less so. As parents we must protect our children from interference with the natural healing mechanism of emotional expression. Society at large and too many parents still confuse the hurt (e.g., loss of a toy) with the emotional discharge or release of the hurt, in this case by crying or tantrums. Some parents try to teach their children that crying is bad since it accomplishes nothing, and may even shame a

child for crying. The truth is that even well-intentioned efforts to soothe or distract a child from crying, though perhaps successful and even necessary at times of stress, is harmful in the long run. Our children recover from hurt and loss by crying, from frustration and insult by tantrums or storming and from frightful experiences by shaking, trembling and sweating. The parents' job is to stay close and help them with their hard feelings. An added value is the blessed knowledge that they do not have to go through the hard times alone.

...*the trauma of condescension*. This is related to "adultism", but specific to the common degrading and debilitating practice of treating children as cutely inadequate, and minimizing or underestimating their enormous intelligence. Adults tend to confuse lack of information and experience with lack of intelligence. To patronize children is an enormous insult. To deny them useful information about how the world works is a great disservice that sets them up for failure. Similarly, to deny them the opportunity to be useful is also a disservice. Parents must ensure that children are given regular opportunities to make real, meaningful contributions to family and community life.

...*the trauma of chronic hopelessness*. Many adults in our society experience chronic hopelessness or apathy. This is a persistent feeling that things are hopeless, that one cannot

make a difference and that it is useless to even try. Excitement and enthusiasm, like passionate outrage, are seen as the stuff of naive childhood, or perhaps as possibilities for remarkable others, but not oneself. While the world is indeed a mess in many ways, the feeling of
chronic hopelessness is nothing but a mental and emotional distress recording left over from the early experiences of being hurt without help or recourse to healing. It is vital that parents challenge this pattern in themselves in order to convey a more realistic and positive attitude to their children. Diane Shisk, an international leader in the Re-evaluation Counselling Community, recommends that the following message be frequently relayed to our children: "There are many problems to be solved. Many people are hurt and unable to treat each other well. But many people are thinking about what should be done to fix things and are joining together to make things right. We will be able to set everything right, and you will be able to help us."

...*the trauma of competition.* This is another very significant reason that primary values of Western Civilisation are doomed to failure. The truth, substantiated by considerable research, is that we do better on all levels (including learning, performance and productivity) when we act with one another in the spirit of cooperation. We need to model and support our children so that they will take delight in and celebrate the success of others, and accept and understand the value and necessity of making mistakes.

...the trauma of militarism. Our society invests a prodigious amount of its available resources in war-making endeavours, sacrificing the real human needs of its people even in times of apparent peace. The propaganda and practices emphasizing violence as the ultimate solution to life's challenges and conflicts can be overwhelming. Conscious parenting must be thoughtful and
persistent in contradicting this conditioning to violence, and providing young people with the information and attitudes necessary to contribute toward a world without war. The rapidly growing prison industry is a related place where more and more children's lives are being sacrificed; this institution of chronic hopelessness and retributive justice must also be challenged.

...the trauma of unnecessary medical interventions. Iatrogenic (medically-induced) illness is almost a household term today. Examples include problems caused by medicalized birth, unnecessary antibiotic use, unnecessary suppression of fever, and vaccine reactions. The common cycle of antibiotic use and tubes for the inner ear for recurrent ear infections, when nutritional changes, such as elimination of dairy produces, would solve the problem in most instances, is a specific example.

...*the trauma of psychiatric drugs.* It is a national shame and disgrace that an estimated 8,000,000 school-age children in the United States are on toxic psychiatric drugs, all for alleged illnesses that are scientifically unproven. This is a social and medical scandal that should disabuse all conscious parents of any remaining illusion that it is safe to blindly trust medical or educational authorities.

...*the trauma of compulsory factory schooling.* Everyone should read the works of John Taylor Gatto, the most informed, thorough and eloquent writer on the subject of education today, to learn about the enormous problems of our compulsory education system. His advice to parents, after 30 years of public school teaching and twice New York State teacher of the year, is as follows: "Breaking the hold of fear on your life is the necessary first step. If you can keep your kid out of any part of the school sequence at all, *keep him or her out of kindergarten*, then first, then second, and maybe third grade. Home-school them at least that far through the zone where most of the damage is done." (Gatto, 2001) If you can't do that, I have two pieces of advice. First, stay close to your children, be their vigorous ally, and let them know that you and they together will figure things out and have great success. Second, protect them against taking on shame from the inevitable experiences that something is wrong when the imposed schedule and structure of school inexorably and routinely violates the self-directed learning tendencies and styles of your children. Let them know, at whatever level they are capable of, that when this happens it is not because they are wrong or inadequate or defective. Rather, explain to them that the schools have some problems, but that you and your children working together will be able to figure out a way to solve these problems. Whatever happens, don't let the spirit of your child be crushed by debilitating shame.

...the trauma of illiteracy and labels such as learning disabled (LD) and attention deficit hyperactivity disorder (ADHD). It is an ongoing shame that the literacy rate of Americans has systematically declined with increased governmental funding and control of education. Learning to read is not a great mystery. The average 5-year-old can master all of the 70 phonograms for reading in six weeks, and is then able to read just about anything. Understanding, of course, comes later. There are methods available to help children who missed the so-called pre-reading skills. It is regrettable that the schools are not doing the job. Even more regrettable is that they blame the children, label them as defective, remove them from their peers, and give them drugs. Parents must protect children from such assaults, and make sure that their children get the support necessary to grow up without stigmatization and without being identified as defective.

...the trauma of a flawed view of human nature.
The harmful practices of our civilization are rooted
in a grievous misunderstanding of human nature.
The schools are designed on the assumption that
there are 'dumb' children, and that children are
like empty machines needing to be programmed
and filled. Punitive, shame-based or controlling
child-rearing practices are legacies of old
fashioned fundamentalist views of fallen, sinful
human nature. Our greedy, profit-driven,
militarist, consumerist culture is based on a view
of human nature without soul or spirit. Psychiatry
is based on a worldview that reduces human
beings and human experience to biology and
chemistry. All of this is motivated by fear that
flawed human nature will win out or, to use the
Darwinian metaphor, that we will be eaten before
we can eat. I believe that human nature, at its
deepest level, is benign and wonderful, that we
are inherently intelligent, resourceful, zestful,
affectionate and relational. By protecting our
children from harm and cynicism, by giving them
accurate information at a level they can
comprehend, and by allowing and encouraging
them to express the pain associated with the hurts
they do suffer, this true nature will blossom.
Perhaps the greatest gifts we can give to our
children are to see them through the eyes of
delight, and to be with them in an attitude of
relaxed confidence that they are turning out well.

*...the trauma of parents unwilling to face their own
traumas.* Perhaps the most fundamental law of

parenting is that we are forced to face the places where it is hard for us to remain thoughtful and loving about our children. We parents have to choose, again and again, between personal transformation on the one hand, and suppressing our children on the other. The main reason we punish or reject our children is because pain associated with our own past traumas is upon us and we are unable or unwilling to face ourselves and take personal responsibility for our state of mind. There are no bad or disgusting or hopeless children, only children who are having a hard time and need loving attention and support. Giving this to them requires facing our own issues, and sometimes getting help for ourselves, in order to come back into a thoughtful and positive place about both ourselves and our children. The alternative is to shut them down and stifle the process of growth.

The Commitment

A commitment to the attitudes embodied in this manifesto means something like this: I recognise that our society is seriously troubled disturbed and dangerous to the well-being of my children and my family in many ways. I also recognise, however, the glorious true nature of my self and my children; therefore, I have complete confidence that my children will develop into happy, creative, and productive adults. I will not blame my children for how I feel. I will take full responsibility for my actions and my state of mind. I am willing to change and continue growing up throughout all of my parenting life. I promise to remain close and affectionate with my children for the rest of my-life.

BOOK 2

Eyes Wide Open: A Second 21st Century Manifesto for Parents

A full three decades ago, at a major university, I learned something in my class on infant psychology. The professor was great—ardent and intelligent, trained at the University of Minnesota Child Development Centre, one of the most prestigious universities in the academic world of child development. He was actively involved in researching infant life and experience. I learned that
newborns could not focus their eyes for a while after birth, a couple of days more or less. I accepted this along with all kinds of other valuable information in my quest to understand life, my own life in particular.

That was 1974. Twelve years later, on August 31, 1986, I learned that my newborn son was intensely focused immediately upon entry from his mother's womb into the world of air—eyes wide open, intense, and appearing angry after a very difficult struggle to get his big head through his mother's cervix. I, too, was wide open after one of the most awesome peak experiences of my life. Eighteen years later, in 2004, I met for the first time another outstanding teacher, and heard a sentence that gave me a clear way to think about this business of focusing infants and other "things I learned at school."

Psychiatrist Thomas Szasz is the finest master of language and logic that I have ever encountered, excelling particularly in the art of creating aphorisms—short, pithy statements of truth. I once heard him speak about his chosen profession, articulating the truth about psychiatry and our so-called mental health system. Dr. Szasz quoted American humorist Josh Billings' quip that, "The problem is not that people don't know anything, it's that they know so many things that ain't so!" (I have later learned from Leonard Roy Frank, editor of *Random House Webster's Quotationary*, that this aphorism more likely came from Artemus Ward, who said that, "It's not so much what folks don't know that causes problems, it's what they do know that ain't so.")

This essay is an effort to answer the question of how people know so much that "ain't so", and live in denial about what is. It is also a sequel to the first manifesto above. As you have read, that piece goes into some detail about our distressed society, and exhorts parents to protect their children from various traumas.
This sequel goes a step further, confronting the fact that however much we are able to protect our individual children from harm, that will not be enough to ensure that they will have a future.

Our world is in peril. Life forms are rapidly being extinguished, the environment is in grave danger of complete collapse, and so is the economy. Billions in our own human species are already suffering, and the continuation of 'our civilization's business as usual' can only have one outcome, and it is an ugly one. Sadly, it is not enough to protect our own children. Unless we demand and create significant change at the level of our civilization, even our own loved and privileged children, and almost definitely our children's children will not survive. Certainly, they will experience a world of overwhelming toxicity and underwhelming biodiversity. The details to back up this sentence are readily available in abundant scientific descriptions for those with eyes to see. This essay explores the psychology of denial and expresses a call to action on behalf of our own and all future generations.

On Seeing

I had another great teacher for a few years. His name was Russell Nees, and he was a remarkable man—a small town Texas minister for decades with an active and involved congregation, moving Christianity forward from fundamentalism to a living experience that God is love, and let your yea mean yes and your nay mean no, and other simple teachings of how to live a conscious, caring life. In his later years, after his wife had died of cancer, Russell was part of a very small group that founded the Optimal Health Centre, a raw food and juice fasting health spa, outside Austin, Texas. One of Russell's greatest pleasures in life was to find what he called white crows, the notion being that one white crow disproved the notion that all crows are black. One person who could see at a distance, for example, or read the history of a place from a rock, showed that seeing was not strictly a function of our physical visual sensory apparatus, operating in present time. Why do you think it was taught that infants couldn't focus? Was my son, Eric, a white crow? He was to me, for sure, but I think it had more to do with the fact that the science of child developmental psychology was seriously establishing itself about the time I was born, which was 1952. Part of that scientific process was to establish norms. Child psychologists are very big on defining average, expected trends in the development of body, mind and behaviour.

The upside of this basic notion is that we are encouraged not to have unrealistic expectations for our children, as in not expecting a baby to understand the logic of conservation of energy. The downside is reflected in rigid age graded segregation and the ubiquitous labelling of children as developmentally delayed and learning disabled because they do not read by age six. There is another huge problem with the establishment of norms. Simply put, it is that normal is not necessarily natural. During the Inquisition, it was normal to persecute women because "everyone knew" (at least everyone in power knew) that they were heretics. In Nazi Germany, it was normal to persecute Jews because "everyone knew" they were an inferior race. Today, it is normal for 15-20% of our children to take psychotropic drugs of one kind or another because "everyone knows" ADHD children need stimulant drugs, and depression is a chemical imbalance requiring antidepressant drugs.

How did it get to be normal for 1 out of 5 people to suffer from a biological or genetic defects that cause them to be failures in social adjustment? Someone has observed children and decided that the norm is to sit quietly and do your homework, and that to do otherwise is abnormal. The question of why this "abnormal" behaviour is interpreted as a biological defect is another vitally important subject which many writers, including myself in all my books, cover in depth. Pertinent here, though, is to notice where the norm of sitting quietly and doing homework was established. It was in the public school classroom! If you have already considered, perhaps with the tutelage of the best current teacher on the subject, John Taylor Gatto, that the design of our educational system is highly oppressive and violating of children's true natures, then you know that these norms are invalid, that they do not reflect the natural development of children, but instead reflect something about the process of adjustment (or not) to oppression.

Do you see the underlying principle here? Norms, whether scientific or simply the values and beliefs that we all hold as a result of what we have learned and therefore think we know, are developed in a context—a certain time, place and social structure or design. The teaching here might be as follows:

Before using norms to make conclusions or decide about actions, it would be best to find out all you can about the development of those norms---the time and place of their establishment, the design of the environment in which the observations were made, the various inputs into the lives of those for whom the norms were being developed, and perhaps most importantly the assumptions, goals and intentions of the environmental designers.

Before you read on, take a minute and apply these principles to the question of infants being able to focus and Eric's value as a white crow. What do you know about the time and place of childbirth in 1952 in the United States? What was its design? What were the various inputs into a newborn's life? What were the assumptions, goals and intentions of the designers of the environment of childbirth in 1952 in the United States?

Here are a few related teachings:

Norms function as expectations and we tend to accept them as given conditions of our world.

Natural and normal are very different concepts. In distressed societies, they rarely coincide.

What we assume to be normal very often reveals little about what is natural.
Our norms generally tell us more about our structures than they do about our natures.

What we think we know is often false.

Once you have the data, the answer is very simple. Common practices of childbirth in 1952 were horrific. The mothers were generally on drugs. My mother was totally unconscious from general anaesthesia; I was on drugs when I was born. It was also common practice to inject a very painful and vision blurring solution into the newborn's eyes immediately after birth. The rest of the picture is equally harsh and upsetting. It is easy to see why infant developmental norms in general would be unnatural, and specifically why infants could not focus.

The bigger teaching:
Our true nature is eyes wide open.

Another vital truth to understand:
We are enormously vulnerable to conditioning.

Most life forms have a very short dependency period, fully mature within hours or days or weeks or at most, as in large mammals, two or three years. Humans, on the other hand, take at least until age 25 or so to fully develop on just a physical level. The brain continues to grow and develop throughout adolescence and into young adulthood. While it is not true, as classical behaviourism states, that we are a blank slate, it is true that we are enormously plastic, dependent and vulnerable to the effects of conditioning.

In fact, our psychological self is not inborn, but develops via the process of internalizing images and experiences that originally occur in our outer lives. Though fortunately limited by our inherent natural tendencies, to a large extent we psychologically become a faithful recording of our environment. This is the basis of much modern psychological theory, but it is not a new idea, and is best understood in classic poems such as this one by Dorothy Lawe Holt:

If A Child

If a child lives with criticism, he learns to condemn.
If a child lives with hostility, he learns to fight.
If a child lives with ridicule, he learns to be shy.
If a child lives with fear, he learns to be
apprehensive.
If a child lives with shame, he learns to feel guilty.

But

If a child lives with tolerance, he learns to be
patient.
If a child lives with encouragement, he learns to
be confident.
If a child lives with acceptance, he learns to love.
If a child lives with approval, he learns to like
himself.
If a child lives with recognition, he learns it is good
to have a goal.
If a child lives with honesty, he learns what truth
is.
If a child lives with fairness, he learns justice.
If a child lives with security, he learns to have faith
in himself and those about him.
If a child lives with friendliness, he learns the world
is a nice place in which to live, to love and be
loved.

It is actually much easier to facilitate the loving qualities because that is our natural bent.

It takes more of a systematic process of hurting and depriving children to install oppressive patterns. Once installed, though, it is relatively easy to trigger those patterns and keep them activated. The primary dynamic is really very simple. It is to make the being afraid, making sure she knows that her survival depends on avoiding the wrath or abandonment of the person on whom her life depends. The end result is very simple: AUTHORITY = TERROR.

The ideal in a culture such as ours that frowns on overt harsh abuse and cowering, whimpering dependents, is to make a child (or citizen) not so fearful that they utterly collapse and cringe, but just fearful enough that they survive reasonably in tact, but are very "respectful" and OBEDIENT to their elders or other authorities. Of course, in our own United States society, it has become increasingly acceptable to collapse and cringe because the medical psychiatric priesthood has afforded a safe explanation for such pathetic behaviour. Do you know what I am talking about here? Think for a moment. What is the usual dynamic when a child or adult exhibits fear, mild or intense? Think about how fear manifests itself. In extreme instances, it involves cringing, tightening, going cold, shaking, trembling, running, screaming, shutting down, agitation, panic, racing thoughts, frequent urination, stress diarrhea, heart racing, elevated blood pressure, insomnia, etc. Milder forms include worry, restlessness, tension, etc.

Let me clarify using the Diagnostic and Statistical Manual of the American Psychiatric Association.

ADHD—difficulty sustaining attention, forgetful, fidgeting, squirming, "driven by a motor."

Bipolar Disorder—pressure to keep talking, thoughts are racing, psychomotor agitation.

Anxiety Disorder—excessive worry, inability to relax.

Panic Disorder—trembling, shaking, fears of…whatever.

I call this the awesome magic trick of so-called biological psychiatry. Despite the complete lack of objective proof that any problem routinely diagnosed as a "mental illness" by a psychiatrist is caused by an existing physical or chemical abnormality, biopsychiatry has transformed socially "unacceptable" expressions of mood and behaviour into medical illnesses, allegedly caused by biological or genetic defects, and treatable with psychotropic drugs or electroshock. All responsibility by psychiatrists is avoided, along with any questions about relational dynamics and social justice issues. In legal terms, all are afforded the protection of "plausible deniability."

A Primer on Conditioning

Installing patterns of fear and more or less blind obedience, though a lot more trouble than supporting our natural bent toward self-determination with eyes wide open, is not all that hard. John Taylor Gatto (2001) does perhaps the best job laying out how this works in our educational system, modelled after a Prussian (German) design that was found effective in creating properly
obedient soldiers and factory workers.

Consider the following two assertions.

Our nature is eyes wide open, brilliantly intelligent, intensely relational in a loving way, and energetically zestful, and inclined toward loving.

Western Civilization, especially as embodied in the current United States of America, is the most destructive civilization in the history of the world.

If you agree with the first statement, then, like me, you try to figure out how it happened that so many of us act in such stupid and mean-spirited ways that untold unnecessary suffering prevails, and the very future of our existence on this planet is in peril. If you disagree, then you can ascribe such horrors to human nature, likely including the ubiquitous presence of alleged biopsychiatric defects in millions of 'mentally ill' people.

If you agree with the second, you try even harder to understand, and you are denied the luxury of the notion that "yes it is bad, but at least our country is a hopeful beacon of light in a dark world." Instead, the task of self-scrutiny and self-inquiry becomes especially demanding and intense.

If you disagree that the United States embodies the most destructive civilization in history, so be it. Perhaps you can agree that it is very destructive. If not, I would encourage you to at least take notice of the reactions that such a statement evokes inside of you. Suffice it to say that billions are suffering unnecessarily. That the inequalities are becoming more and more glaring all the time, that myriad life forms are rapidly being extinguished, that our economic environment is dangerously shaky and our natural web of existence is in grievous peril. These are facts to those with eyes can see. A fundamentalist might see them and attest to their inevitability as prophesied.

Count me among those who see the consequences of human choice and action. My purpose just now is simply to say that, because of our enormous vulnerability to conditioning, it is very possible to override and distort our natural intelligent and loving tendencies, and create patterns in people that are based in fear and denial, to move people from eyes wide open to eyes tightly shut. The best writer I know on this process is Derrick Jensen, in his books, *A Language Older Than Words,* and *The Culture of Make Believe.*

From Eyes Wide Open to A Culture of Denial: An Awful Transmutation

As noted above, it is relatively easy to make children fearful and inclined to obedience. There is a great deal of writing on the psychological dynamics of conditioning children, all my own books included. The interested reader may refer to these sources. Just now, I want to point out one particular effect, reflected in the following teaching:

We see the world not as it is, but as we are.

Perception seems to duplicate what is out there as when we all see a chair or bird or whatever. That is only the surface of things, however, and even then, it is very unreliable, as evidenced for example in eyewitness testimony in criminal trials. It is even worse for entirely subjective phenomenon like so-called mental illness.

The provocative movie "What the Bleep Do We Know?" (2004) shows interviews with quantum physicists and other consciousness researchers and reveals some of the dilemmas involved in the perceptual process. For example, an inner image evokes the same physiological and sensory dynamics as an outer image; simply imagining something creates a similar effect to actually seeing it. Further, we are often unable to see something for which we have no inner category or reference point.

My introductory psychology textbook tells the story of pygmy man named Kenge who is with a white anthropologist who points out a creature way out across a large open space. Kenge sees an insect, and then the anthropologist drives him toward the insect, which gets increasingly larger as Kenge shows evidence of building fear and confusion. Eventually he recognizes a buffalo, and is awed that the insect tuned into a buffalo. The text explains that Kenge lived his whole life in a jungle where there were no large open distances and therefore his brain and visual apparatus had not learned to compensate for distance the way one does when experienced with open spaces.

"What the Bleep Do We Know" recounts the story of Columbus's arrival in the West Indies. The native Arawak Indians who met the men who came ashore literally could not see the ships that brought them. Eventually they were able to after one man figured it out and "saw" the ships. The idea was that they had no category, no inner schema, and therefore could not configure the perception. Whether or not this story has a factual basis, it reveals a deep truth that we witness all the time.

We tend not to see things that we have not experienced, or do not expect.

Have you ever walked with someone who knows all about the plant or animal life in a given area?

Have you had the experience of having pointed out to you the presence of some creature that you literally could not see? My sister was once walking with a guide in the Costa Rican jungle, and despite warnings about the deadly vipers, she came within a hair of putting her hand on one that she did not "see," could not "see." Her guide could see all kinds of things in the jungle that the tourists could not see. Perhaps you have heard that Eskimos have 20 words for snow. How much differentiation do you make between different types of snowflakes? Do you "see" the different types? How often do we overlook the unexpected? How often do we overlook or dismiss the island of clarity in someone diagnosed as a "schizophrenic psychotic?" Conversely,

*We tend to see things that we expect **or need** to see, even when they are not there.*

Consider Daniel Rosenhan's (1973) famous experiment in which eight totally sane "pseudo-patients", mostly professional people, gained secret admission to different mental hospitals by falsely complaining that they had been hearing voices over the past three weeks mentioning the words "empty," "hollow," and "thud." No other psychological abnormalities were related or discovered in the psychological intake exams. All eight pseudo-patients were admitted, all as "schizophrenic," except for one "manic-depressive." After gaining admission, each person acted totally sane, and each said that the voices had disappeared. Each patient asked frequently about discharge plans. The length of hospitalizations ranged from 7 to 52 days (averaging 19 days). Attendants only came outside the "cage" (the nursing station) 11.5 times per shift. Psychiatrists rarely interacted meaningfully with the pseudo-patients. Discharge diagnoses were all "schizophrenia, in remission." Most of the other "real" patients knew for certain that the pseudo-patients were faking, but none of the professional staff suspected that reality. A follow-up study was then done in a research and teaching hospital whose staff had heard about the previous study. The staff were warned that in the next three months there would be one or more pseudo-patients attempting to be admitted to their hospital. Importantly, *no actual pseudopatients even attempted admission.*

Among the 193 patients admitted for psychiatric treatment during this three-month period, 41 genuine patients were suspected, with high confidence, of being pseudo-patients by at least one member of the staff. Twenty-three were considered suspect by a psychiatrist. Both a psychiatrist and one other staff member suspected 19. This experiment clearly shows the effect of beliefs on perception and action. Classic educational research has revealed how one can actually affect others through their beliefs and attitudes. This is often called the self-fulfilling prophecy. Otherwise known as the Pygmalion effect, it might better be called the other-fulfilling prophecy. *Others tend to live up (or down) to the images we hold for them.*

Have you heard of the Pygmalion effect? The name comes from George Bernard Shaw's play "Pygmalion," in which Professor Henry Higgins claims he can take a Cockney flower girl and pass her off as a Duchess. He succeeds via rigorous retraining, of which the most important element has to do with the effect of altered images and expectations. The girl, Eliza Doolittle, points out in a comment to her trainee, Higgins' friend Pickering that anyone can learn the dress and manner, but that "the difference between a lady and a flower girl is not in how she behaves but in how she is treated. I shall always be a flower girl to Professor Higgins, because he treats me as a flower girl, and always will, but I know I can be a lady to you because you always treat me as a lady, and always will."

There has been considerable educational research showing that teacher expectations have a dramatic effect on student learning and performance.
(http://www.ncrel.org/sdrs/areas/issues/educatrs/leadrshp/le0bam.htm.)
As an example, Rosenthal and Jacobson (1968) administered IQ tests to children aged six-to-twelve years, all drawn from the same school. The children were assigned either to an experimental group or a control group. When teachers were told

that the children in the experimental group were "high achievers", these children showed significant IQ gains compared with the children in the control group over the course of one year, despite the fact that allocation to each group had been random. Business consultants tend to best summarise the process:

1) We form certain expectations of people and events.
2) We communicate those expectations with certain cues.
3) People tend to respond to these cues by adjusting their behaviour to match.
4) The result is that the original expectations come true.
(http://www.accel-team.com/pygmalion/prophecy_01.html)

These four points clearly convey the interacting dynamic. However, I want to emphasize a related point, which is that our inner images and expectations not only affect what we communicate; as in the above stories of Kenge and the Arawak Indians, they actually tend to determine what we see and therefore can communicate.

We tend not to see anything, even in plain sight, that threatens our conditioned beliefs and values.

Consider the following excerpt from an interview of David Edwards, the author of *Burning All Illusions*, by Derrick Jensen:

> "In a study conducted in the 1960s] a man by the name of Lester Luborsky used a special camera to track the eye movements of people who were asked to look at a set of pictures, three of which involved sexual images. One, for example, showed a woman's breast, beyond which could be seen a man reading a newspaper. The results were amazing. Many viewers were able to avoid letting their gaze stray even once to the sexually suggestive parts of the pictures, and later, when asked to describe the content of the pictures, they remembered little or nothing suggestive about them. Some people couldn't even recall having seen those three pictures at all.
>
> "What interests me is that, in order to avoid looking at the objectionable parts of the pictures, those people had to know in some part of their minds what the picture contained so that they could know to avoid it. In other words, when the mind detects something offensive or threatening to our worldview, it somehow deflects our awareness. This avoidance system is incredibly efficient. We know exactly where not to look." (*SUN* magazine, June 2000)

The best explanation I know for this dynamic is that we humans have a natural self-protective tendency to shield ourselves from the memory and effects of hurtful or threatening experiences.

Such protection easily becomes convenient as we justify our ways and attitudes, and rationalize our fears, doubts, hesitancies and uncertainties. This may be best described by people like psychiatrist Alice Miller, in describing the cycle of child abuse. An abused child internalizes that abuse, and then represses it in order to function without overwhelming feelings of hurt, fear and shame, only to have these very feelings re-stimulated years later as an adult in the face of his or her own children. As Miller says, "It is a tragic fact that parents beat their own children in order to escape the feelings stemming from how they were treated by their own parents." In any event, the dynamics of denial are there, and huge numbers of our citizens blindly accept, allow, and promote the current inequities, injustices, and ravages of our existence on this planet.

What may for each individual have been at one point a very necessary self-protective survival dynamic now becomes blind denial that lends to avoiding and perpetuating the destructive actions that hamper our relationships and even endanger our existence.

The age-old "Emperor Who Has No Clothes" lives in this moment. Some people are able to see his nakedness and point it out, some see it and are too beaten down to say anything, and very many are in such apathy or absorbed short-term selfish interest that they care not to even look, or perhaps they see magnificent clothing where it does not exist. In any event, our children are in peril.

Denial, Oppression, and Claims to Virtue

We have briefly examined the mechanisms of denial. We have acknowledged its protective function, and suggested that such protection becomes counterproductive when it is locked in as a conditioned pattern unrelated to present time reality, a time bomb just waiting to be activated, a rigid ideology or attitude that brooks little if any contradiction. This divorce from present reality for the sake of defending internalized beliefs, ideas, and patterns means that defence of same becomes more important than the best interests or highest good of life. Such denial and defence of false selves is the major psychological force that drives cruelty, injustice, indifference and all forms of irrationality. It is the psychological engine of the systematic mistreatment that we call oppression, and the blatant disregard of all life forms that we see in world structures today.

A huge key in understanding the reality and dynamics of oppression is the concept of claims to virtue. It seems that every cruelty, every injustice, every disregard of the best interests of life has a claim to virtue. There is always some justification, some reason that this injustice, this destruction, this killing, this extinction, this war, this soul murder is not only necessary, but maybe even a good thing. Here are some examples that come to mind. We have all heard the mantra called, "Better safe than sorry." As with most claims to virtue, this one has some truth in it—might be a better idea not to dive off that 40 foot cliff given you have not plumbed the depths of the water below. On the other hand, one of my daughter's summer vacation highlights was her leap off of that 40-foot cliff! The relevant point here is that the nature of life is uncertainty; without risk, we live in inertia and apathy. We choose to be safe and stay at home instead of asking for a date or starting a new project, or speaking out at the legislature, or exploring that wild zone.

I was at a small conference recently, called "The Origins of Love and Violence." The featured speaker was Suzanne Arms, still going strong over 30 years after her breakthrough book, *Immaculate Deception,* started a social movement to reclaim the beautiful wonders of natural childbirth for mothers and babies from the clutches of technological control. The claim to virtue is "better safe than sorry," that birth is painful and difficult, and that we have all this great technology to make it safe. Suzanne Arms describes the reality even today:

> "Women continue to be denied access to alternatives to routine and standard approaches to birth that have no basis in scientific evidence and which dis-empower and hurt themselves and their babies. I watch with pain in my heart as the level of fear among childbearing women, birth professionals and young people grows and

the public's passivity and numbness about birth deepens.   I am deeply concerned that technology and aggressive medical management now dominate most births in the industrialized world and reshape birth in urban areas in much the rest of the world. Even in Greece, Mexico and the island of Bali, induced labour, drugs, episiotomies, vacuum extraction, caesarean, and the forced separation of babies from their mothers right after birth have become the norm, and haemorrhage, infection, birth trauma and bottle feeding follow."
(www.birthingthefuture.com)

As with all efforts to sort out the conflicting views and approach the truth, one has to do some work, go beyond obvious sources which tend to parrot the mainstream beliefs, be willing to face our own possible false beliefs or illusions, and come to our own conclusions. I recommend Suzanne Arms' books and website as one source of data. My own reading and experience tells me it is true that home birth and midwives are generally safer than hospital birth, and that the prenatal and perinatal experience provides the foundation of our being. The premise of that conference, that the origins of love and violence, lie in the experiences of babies and others before, during and after birth, holds great truth.

This passage comes from a pamphlet titled'Birthing the Future', which reads: "MOST of what happens to mothers and babies today—*including* common medical practices and exposure to environmental toxins—harms them or *disrupts* their development." Could this be true? If it is, then that is intense oppression of mothers and babies. Decide for yourself. Here is another seemingly mundane example. How often do children hear "Be Careful!" In fact, is that not the second most ubiquitous mantra of our culture today? (First is "BUY something now.") Terror alert. Terrorist. Child abductor. Job loss. Be afraid. Fear. Fear. Fear. Here is an excerpt on the subject from my own book; *The Wildest Colts Make The Best Horses:*

> There seems to be great confusion in our society about fear. We extol fearlessness, placing great value on the person (generally a man) who "knows no fear." At the same time, we tend to be very fearful and manifest this fear in how we treat our children. I challenge you to notice how often you say "Be careful" to your child. Think about it. Jean Liedloff, in *The Continuum Concept*, gives a wonderful illustration of childrearing in a nature-based tribal society. The children are free to range the edges of steep cliffs and fire pits without concern. They are expected to learn awareness, not caution. In our own society, we teach our children to be afraid. Notice the mailings and late night TV spots depicting lost

children. The impression is that children are in great danger of abduction; yet the actual number of abductions is very small and, in fact, parents who have been denied legal custody commit more than 90 percent of these so-called "abductions". The way mass media handles "News" in this country saturates us with fear. Sensationalist journalism takes a horrific incident from anywhere in the state, country or world and brings it into your home and into your mind. You feel as if these daily horrors were happening right next door and you were indeed living in an extremely dangerous neighbourhood.

The claim to virtue is obvious; we all want to keep our children safe, and there are dangers. I mentioned some above in reference to my 21st Century Manifesto for Parenting. There are no guarantees. Could it be that our frequent admonishments to be careful actually suppress our children's awareness, natural curiosity and exploration by making them fearful and conveying an expectation of harm or failure? You decide, but check yourself out by considering the possibility of enthusiastically telling your daughter to "Take a Risk!" as she heads out the door today.

The New Intrusion Initiative

One other thing to think about as she heads out the door, especially if she is going to school, or to a doctor's appointment, or anywhere that constitutes a physical health check or an interface with a state program. Have you heard of the President's 'New Freedom Commission'? It was set up to make recommendations for our so-called mental health system.

I and others are writing and speaking about the New Freedom recommendations, which call for universal mental health screening; for example, the government wants "access" to all 52 million children and 6 million adults in our public schools. It also wants to make sure a child gets "screened for mental illness" every time they get a health check-up. Think about it. We have nearly 10 million school-age children already on psychotropic drugs in this country. Does that sound like an access problem? The claim to virtue is that we need to find and care for these sick mentally ill children. The truth is that the New Freedom Commission is driven by the same forces that created the Texas Medication Algorithm Project (TMAP). This is a formula which calls for specific drugs for each psychiatric diagnosis. It is mandated by the state mental health system, and it is being spread all over the country. Care to guess who is behind it? Cui bono? Who benefits? The obvious answer, once you know this game, is Big Pharma; the drug companies donated a lot of money to the state to develop this programme, from which they'll reap massive profits because almost every person diagnosed as "mentally ill" will receive a prescription for some psychoactive drug they manufacture.

New Freedom is doublespeak for New Intrusion; access means recruitment, screening means labelling, treating means drugging, service means profit. At its roots, this is a very cynical move for control and profit. The poisonous tree's secondary fruit, after corporate profit, is damaged children.

Psychiatry and Militarism: A World in Peril

Our world is in peril. Do you see what I see? I see the so-called third world in misery, the first world in fear and nonsense. More than one billion souls around the world live in slums. The "free" world is looking more and more like a police state. We live under a so-called Patriot Act, even as the planet is raped and decimated with clear cuts, poisoned air and water, nuclear proliferation and waste, etc. This "free" world is a military aggressor who won't quit till it swallows up the whole world..

Are you one of the many citizens who either celebrate or at the very least support U.S. military aggression? Or are you like Henry David Thoreau who, during the time of slavery, said "My outrage at my country spoils my walk!" Are you completely ashamed and aghast at cruelty and atrocities the United States has inflicted on so many people around the world? Or are you like Senator James Inhofe of Oklahoma and other apologists? During the Senate investigations of the abuse of Iraqi prisoners at Abu Ghraib, Inhofe opined that "I'm probably not the only one up at this table that is more outraged by the outrage than we are by the treatment." How is that for a claim to virtue? He is saying in effect, I am patriotic so I do not judge my country's actions.

Most world citizens have by now at least heard that there is a huge controversy about what actually happened on September 11, 2001, when airplanes were hijacked and buildings toppled in the United States. For those with eyes to see, it is apparent that at the very least, the story of the official 911 Commission is deeply flawed. Many think that rogue elements within our own government had to have played a role to negate U.S. air defense and pull off the events of that day, and to bring those buildings down in a way that looks just like controlled demolition. For those readers interested in the most intelligent analysis I have found of that story, I recommend Webster' Griffin Tarpley's book, *9/11 Synthetic Terror: Made in USA.* At the very least, readers will find that a willingness to take a close look at the possibility that 9/11 was an inside job is a most powerful exercise in the dynamic I am encouraging in this little book: confronting reality head-on, regardless.

Since we are confronting denial in psychiatry and in militarism, it behooves us to take a quick look at the link between these two major sources of oppression. Here is a present time link between the mental health system and the military. I quote BBC News correspondent Matthew Davis: "Authors of a report in the *New England Journal of Medicine* say that since late 2002, psychiatrists and psychologists have been part of a programme designed to increase fear and distress among prisoners as a means to getting intelligence." (6-24-05, http://news.bbc.co.uk/2/hi/americas/4620073.stm)

The concept is called "Biscuit Teams"—behavioural science consultation teams designed to assist interrogators in breaking down prisoners. One result of the Iraq war, consistent with the history of all wars, is the return to the United States
of a great number of psychiatric casualties, soldiers who suffer from what is now called Post Traumatic Stress Disorder (PTSD). The April 20, 2005 edition of the *Fort Hood Herald* has an article by Joshua Cleveland on the PTSD experience among soldiers returning to Fort Hood from the Middle East war zone. Particularly scary is the article's reference to a recent issue of the medical journal, *Science,* in which a certain "Mark Eisenberg and colleagues from the Weismann Institute of Science in Rehovot, Israel, reported that they are closer to selectively wiping out traumatic memories from a person's brain." A major effect of biopsychiatry is to absolve everyone from responsibility. Rather than taking on the hard task of confronting issues of community, social and economic justice, hurt or distressed individuals are labelled as having biological or genetic defects, that is, they are "mentally ill." These Israeli scientists are trying to develop drugs that will wipe out select memories, and Fort Hood is paying attention. This today in our society is an acceptable alternative to confronting the social and economic factors that create and justify the horrors of unnecessary warfare, and accepting full responsibility for the wounded men and women.

It is also a way of avoiding the awful responsibility for unnecessarily making killers of adolescent and young adult men. I recently heard investigative journalist Seymour Hersh on Amy Goodman's *Democracy Now* radio show. Hersh is famous for breaking the story of the My Lai massacre, and for his current work on Afghanistan and Iraq, including breaking the story of the Abu Ghraib tortures. On Goodman's show, Hersh said that 35 years ago he had found the mother of one of the men who participated in the My Lai massacre. The mother's words: "I gave them a good boy. And they sent me back a murderer." Last year, he found the mother of one of the Abu Ghraib soldiers, who found a CD of pictures from Abu Ghraib, pictures that in Hersh's words, "no mother should see." One was published in the *New Yorker*.
(http://www.democracynow.org/article.pl?sid=05/0 1/26/1450204#transcript)

The history of Nazi Germany is frequently invoked as the prime example of military policy driven by psychiatric belief. The principles of eugenics, or improvement of the species via genetic selection, were used to justify the Holocaust. Today, in a less dramatic way than the concentration camps, the same principles justify the New Intrusion initiative, universal mental health screening, and the mass drugging of our nation's children.

On October 4, 2004, the Texas House held a select committee hearing to explore the ubiquitous use of psychotropic drugs on foster children. Dr. Joseph Burkett, medical director for Tarrant County Mental Health Mental Retardation, justified the fact that a high percentage of these children were on several dangerous psychotropic drugs at once, with his testimony that, "A lot of these kids come from bad gene pools." (Mitch Mitchell, "MHMR official regrets 'gene pool' remarks," Fort Worth Star-Telegram, 11-3-04)

Speaking of our children, here is Christian Parenti, from his book, *The Freedom,* on the country's first year in Iraq:

> "I have seen several children in Baghdad with enlarged heads and huge veins bulging from their skulls and been told that this condition and other bizarre cancers and childhood diseases are linked to roughly 17,000 tons of depleted uranium-tipped weaponry that the United States used on Iraq during both wars." The NGO Child Victims of War says that, "the number of Iraqi babies born with serious deformities has risen from 3.04 per thousand in 1991 to 22.19 per thousand in 2001. Babies born with Down Syndrome have increased nearly fivefold and there [has been] a rash of cases of previously little known eye problems." (p 57)

Seeing (or not) the Truth

The list of cruelties, injustices and irrationalities can go on and on, but the relevant point is that, as George Orwell once said, "To see what is in front of one's nose requires a constant struggle." As I write this sentence, the United States Senate is apologizing to the country for persistently blocking anti-lynching legislation during that not so distant period of infamy. At the same time, the Senate unanimously supports more and more weapons and soldiers and death and destruction and money in a pre-emptive mass aggression in Iraq. Why is that? We know the shifting sands of the various claims to virtue, but why is it really? One answer, of course, is about present-time power, oil and money. But why is it so difficult to see the truth? Orwell's statement does not seem to apply to children as much as it does to adults..

Here are R.D. Laing's three rules, from *The Politics of Experience,* on how to live in a world of denial:

Rule A: Don't.
Rule B: Rule A does not exist.
Rule C: Do not discuss the existence or non-existence of Rules A, B, or C.

Don't look at what we are doing and certainly don't question it. This is a free and democratic, peace-loving country. We are happy for you to see exactly what is going on in Iraq and everything about our history and ongoing actions and communications in that region. So leave it alone, and go out to the mall and buy something — anything.

Here is Laing on destroying the ability to see clearly: "In order to rationalize our military-industrial complex, we have to destroy our capacity to see clearly any more what is in front of, and to imagine what is beyond, our noses. Long before a
thermonuclear war can come about, we have had to lay waste our own sanity. We begin with the children. It is imperative to catch them in time. Without the most thorough and rapid brainwashing their dirty minds would see through our dirty tricks. Children are not yet fools, but we shall turn them into imbeciles like ourselves, with high I.Q's if possible." (Derrick Jensen's *Culture of Make Believe,* pp 57-58.)

I don't want to go on ranting about the Iraq horror. My focus here is on how this kind of thing is allowed, supported and justified. My own writings devote time and energy to exposing the false claims to virtue around the unnecessary, extremely harmful and dangerous practices of biological psychiatry, such as drugging literally millions of our precious children with body-damaging, mind-bending, and soul-crushing psychotropic drugs. How is this allowed and accepted? How do people lose the ability to see and to exercise common sense? Much has been written about our educational system by high-minded teachers like John Holt and John Gatto. They have written about how schools are designed to create useful, obedient workers and soldiers. I learned from the poet David Whyte about the derivation of the most important word in the workplace lexicon and in the special language of schools. The word is "management"—good old behaviour management, classroom management, managing children's behaviour. Manager comes from the Old Italian and French words, maneggio and manege, meaning the training, handling and riding of a horse. So here is a paragraph from David Whyte's book, *Crossing the Unknown Sea*:

> "It is strange to think that the whole spirit of management is derived from the image of getting on the back of a beast, digging your knees in, and heading it in a certain direction. The word manager conjures the image of domination, command, and ultimate control, and the taming of a potentially wild energy. It also implies a basic unwillingness on the part of the people to be managed, a force to be corralled and reined in. All appropriate things if you want to ride a horse, but most people don't respond very passionately or creatively to being ridden, and the words giddy up there only go so far in creating the kind of responsible participation we are looking for." (p. 240)

The bad news is management; the good news is inherent wild, free nature. The good news is a wild, diverse planet. The bad news is that our "civilization" is the most destructive ever. Its core values are two: maximum profit and minimum liability. Its fundamental strategies are two: conquest abroad, repression at home. Everything in it is geared toward the commodification and exploitation of life. Trees become board feet of lumber, land a resource to "develop", animals are food products, and children are a product market for anything: electronic
games, candy, massive amounts of psychiatric drugs, etcetera.

Conclusion

I offer no ready solution, but I have five directions:

First is to confront the truth, however hard and whatever the price you must pay. Such confrontation is not likely to bring hope; it's more likely hopelessness. It is absolutely necessary, however, to allow for the possibility of going beyond hope and hopelessness to a simple embrace of reality, and eventually the remotest possibility of real cultural change. Here are some examples of what I mean: If we don't confront the horror of labelling and drugging our children, they go on being labelled and drugged. If we don't confront the tragedy of preemptive war and unnecessary killing and destruction, we go on killing and destroying. If we don't face the wrenching grief that goes with destruction and deterioration of this planet's life and biosphere, then we are destroyed.

Second is to hold onto a vision of what can be. It is important to confront, but it is not enough to only see the horror, or to oppose it. At every level, we must replace false beliefs with true ones, and thoughtless, or despairing visions with those of beauty and reconciliation. As one example, consider my friend Bob Collier's "default visualization," which he developed as his primary asset in "getting around all [his] mental obstacles" to parenting his daughter.

I imagined my daughter's face, as happy as I could make it, and her posture as it would be if she was having fun. Just that. Like a snapshot. I carried that 'snapshot' around in my mind all day, every day, until it became so strong it was always the easiest thing for me to think of and always the general 'blueprint' I was working to. "Things are not brought into being by thinking about their opposites." The visualizing, however, was much more haphazard, although it was relatively easy to imagine good things for my daughter. It was imagining good things for myself that was the real struggle, because of my 'mental blocks' in that respect. I kept my default visualization in my consciousness, adding details to my general vision or to specific 'mini-visions' at various times whenever I was capable of doing so, and I steadfastly practiced using words and phrases that supported continuous forward movement in my daughter's development. That was my core strategy throughout all those years. And it worked beautifully. (Collier, 2003)

In a similar vein, I offer this Universal Declaration of Mental Rights and Freedoms as a wonderful vision:.

We hold this truth,
That all human beings are created different.
That every human being has the right to be mentally free and independent.

That every human being has the right to feel, see, hear, sense, imagine, believe or experience anything at all, in any way, at any time.

That every human being has the right to behave in any way that does not harm others or break fair and just laws.

That no human being shall be subjected without consent to incarceration, restraint, punishment, or psychological or medical intervention in an attempt to control, repress or alter the individual's thoughts, feelings or experiences. (http://adbusters.org/metas/psycho/prozacspotlight/madpridetour/madprideday.html)

Third, we must not only have a vision, but we must know it to be already true. This seems like a great contradiction of the notion of confronting the tragedies and horrors, and feeling the pain that goes with facing suffering. Wayne Dyer, however, taught me a lot about this through his books, notably one title, *You'll see it when you believe it.* Notice how this title playfully turns the popular "I'll believe it when I see it," on its head. Dyer appreciates the perennial spiritual wisdom, which teaches us that creation works from the inside out, beginning with an inner idea or vision, which is later brought into physical form. The teaching is that when you really know it is true inside yourself, and when that knowing includes the power of intention whereby you act on this knowing that it is already true in the spirit, and then it is just a matter of more or less time before it comes into form.

Fourth, in Gandhi's famous words, "Become the change you want to see." It is necessary but not sufficient to see what is. It is necessary but not sufficient to see what can be. It goes even deeper to know this truth already exists in the spirit. From this place comes our intention, and from this intention flows our action. We become that which we envision, and that which we want to see in others and in the world. Become the lesson you would teach. We are speakers of truth, lovers of life, peacemakers, gardeners, ecologists, people who live from a place of reverence for life, in Albert Schweitzer's phrase, "reverence for all life" (1934). We care for our children and about their welfare and we will do all that we can to protect them from harm. All of this is the way we express our love for them.

Finally, there remains a different call to action. We not only live the way we want to live, we insist that the world confront its irrationalities and unnecessarily damaging ways of being. We stand up for the future of our children by standing up to present denial and life-destroying decisions and behaviours. We refuse to be silent; we refuse to cooperate with a civilization that promotes death over life, money over lovingkindness, comfort over justice. Martin Luther King Jr. authored one of my favorite quotes: "Human salvation lies in the hands of the creatively maladjusted" (1963). But one area especially needs concentrated attention because it affects so vitally the interests of our children. We must derail this "New Freedom" horror and help defend and protect our children and families from even more unnecessary labelling and drugging. We are very active and strong. In 2005, we prevented the passage of a bill before the 2005 Texas legislature that would have codified mental health screening policies into law for example, but the psychiatric-pharmaceutical complex is relentless and we have to be ever vigilant.

There is a long and honourable tradition of civil disobedience in this country, reflecting the fact that allegiance to truth trumps obedience to irrational and cruel oppression. Join us in refusing to comply with biopsychiatric intrusion into our children's lives. We have truth and deep passion on our side. Have you ever noticed the great value placed on being nice? Perhaps, like me, you heard your mother say, perhaps many times, "If you can't say anything nice, don't say anything at all." Maybe you heard someone tell a child in an effort to shame and control him: "You're behaving like an animal!" Just now, when civilization is on a forced march to its ruin, being nice is not fitting. I suggest replacing this admonition with the following: "Stop acting like a civilized human being!" To paraphrase a line from one of Robbie Robertson's song, "Let's make a noise in this world!"

REFERENCES

Breeding, J. *The Wildest Colts Make the Best Horses,* Austin, TX: GW & Co., 2002.

Breeding, J. *True Nature and Great Misunderstandings: How We Care For Our Children According To Our Understanding.* [CITY:?] Eakin Press, 2003.

Breeding, J. *The Necessity Of Madness And Unproductivity: Psychiatric Oppression Or Human Transformation.* London: Chipmunka Press, 2003.

Collier, B. *Parental Intelligence.* (2004) Ebook may be downloaded at Bob's website, www.parental-intelligence.com.

Gatto, J. *The Underground History of American Education.* NY: Oxford Village Press, 2001, pp 303 1nd 306 (See www.johntaylorgatto.com).

Jensen, D. *A Language Older Than Words.* NY: Context Books, 2000.

King, M.L. Jr., *Strength to Love*, NY: Harper & Row, p. 17, 1963]

Laing, R.D. *The Politics of Experience. NY: Penguin Books, 1967.*

Parenti, C. *The Freedom. NY: The New Press, 2004.*

Rosenhan, D. L. *"On Being Sane In Insane Places."* Science, 1973, Vol. 179, p. 250 – 258.

Schweitzer, A."Religion and Modern Civilization" (pt. 2), Christian Century, 28 November 1934.

Whyte, D. *Crossing the Unknown Sea*. NY: Berkeley Publishing, 2001.

Note

1. See investigative reporter Nanci Wilson's series as a starting point to learn about this growing scandal; a good place to start is her 9-30-04 piece at http://keyetv.com/investigativevideo/?cat=10&next=10. Also see the British Medical Journal series by Jeanne Lenzer; you might start with her 6-19-04 article (http://www.underreported.com/modules.php?op=modload&name=News&file=article&sid=1328&mode=thread&order=0&thold=0). Also see our Declaration of Refusal to Comply (http://www.ablechild.org/declaration%20of%20refusal.aspx).

About the Author

John Breeding, Ph.D., is a psychologist with a private counselling practice in Austin, Texas. A significant part of his work involves counselling parents and children. He lectures and leads workshops for parents and educators especially on handling the challenges of a child who has been psychiatrically labeled. He is director of Wildest Colts Resources, a non-profit organization whose purpose is to assist adults in becoming more effective in their work with young people, offering non-drug alternatives to helping young people who are having a hard time. He is also director of Texans For Safe Education, a citizens group dedicated to challenging the ever-increasing role of psychiatry and psychiatric drugs in the schools. Dr. Breeding is also active in other struggles against psychiatric oppression, including the psychiatric drugging of elders in nursing homes.

Dr. Breeding has also been active for over a decade in challenging the psychiatric practice of electroshock. For many years, he served on the advisory board of the World Association of Electroshock Survivors and was instrumental in the passage of significant legislation regulating electroshock and providing protection for Texas citizens regarding the use of electroshock. He is a founding member of the Coalition for the Abolition of Electroshock in Texas (CAEST). (www.endofshock.com)

Dr. Breeding was born in 1952 and obtained his doctorate in school psychology from the University of Texas in 1983. He is the author of three other books: *The Wildest Colts Make the Best Horses, The Necessity of Madness and Unproductivity: Psychiatric Oppression or Human Transformation,* and *True Nature and Great Misunderstandings.* He is also the father of two children, Eric and Vanessa, and a stepson, Gardiner. His website can be viewed at www.wildestcolts.com.

www.ingramcontent.com/pod-product-compliance
Lightning Source LLC
Chambersburg PA
CBHW031219270326
41931CB00006B/615